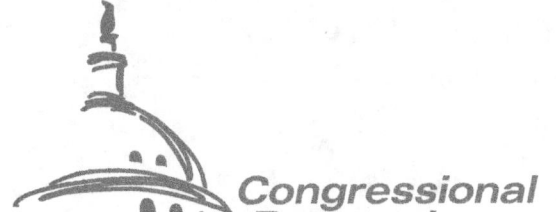

Laws Affecting the Federal Employees Health Benefits Program (FEHBP)

Annie L. Mach
Analyst in Health Care Financing

Ada S. Cornell
Information Research Specialist

September 19, 2012

Congressional Research Service
7-5700
www.crs.gov
R42741

CRS Report for Congress
Prepared for Members and Committees of Congress

Summary

The Federal Employees Health Benefits Program (FEHBP) has been in existence for over 50 years. Since its creation, it has provided private health insurance coverage to federal employees, annuitants, and their dependents. It is the largest employer-sponsored health insurance program in the country; in 2010, nearly 8 million individuals were covered under FEHBP.

The program was created by the Federal Employees Health Benefits Act of 1959 (FEHBA, P.L. 86-382). FEHBA and its subsequent amendments established the parameters for eligibility and the election of coverage; the types of health plans and benefits that may be offered; the level of the government's share of premiums; the Employees Health Benefits Fund to pay for program expenses; and provisions for studies, reports, and audits. FEHBA also outlined the role of the Office of Personnel Management (OPM). By law, OPM is given the authority to contract with insurers and to prescribe regulations to manage FEHBP, among other duties.

The general model of FEHBP has not changed since its inception in 1959. FEHBP was and is a program that allows competing private insurers to offer numerous types of coverage to enrollees within broad federal guidelines. The federal government and the employee/annuitant have always shared the cost of the premium, and generally, employees and annuitants have always had access to the same plans at the same cost. However, specific features of FEHBP have been modified, in some cases multiple times, by Congress and OPM. For example, eligibility has been expanded to include additional types of federal employees and dependents, the formula for determining the government's share of premiums has changed, and the types of health benefits offered through FEHBP plans have been broadened.

Congressional policymakers share responsibility with OPM for the program's viability and sustainability. Congress has financial and administrative interest in the program, as the government pays for a share of FEHBP premiums and Congress has legislative authority to modify FEHBP. Congressional interest in FEHBP also extends to FEHBP's potential applicability as a model for other health care programs or as an avenue to provide coverage, such as extending aspects of FEHBP to Medicare, or using it as one of the models for the state exchanges under the Patient Protection and Affordable Care Act (ACA, P.L. 111-148, as amended).

The purpose of the report is to provide historical and background information that helps explain how FEHBP has evolved into the program it is today. Policymakers may use this report to understand how Congress has interacted with FEHBP in the past, and to inform its future interactions with FEHBP. Specifically, the report includes short discussions of how Congress has effected and maintained policy changes to FEHBP by restricting the use of federal funds; changed the formula for determining the government's share of FEHBP premiums; expanded eligibility for the program; and implemented policies that affect the relationship between Medicare and FEHBP. The **Appendix** includes detailed summaries of selected laws or provisions of laws that have directly amended or otherwise changed FEHBP.

Contents

Introduction 1
    Interest in FEHBP 2
    Scope of Report 3
Conditions on FEHBP Use of Federal Funds 4
Premium Determinations 5
Eligibility 7
Medicare and FEHBP 11

Tables

Table 1. Provisions of Laws Conditioning the Use of Federal Funds for FEHBP 5
Table 2. Provisions of Laws Related to Changes in How the Government's Share of the
    Premium Is Determined 6
Table 3. Laws Affecting Eligibility for FEHBP 8
Table 4. Provisions Related to Changing How FEHBP and Medicare Interact 12

Appendixes

Appendix. FEHBP Legislative History 13

Contacts

Author Contact Information 39

Introduction

The Federal Employees Health Benefits program (FEHBP) provides private health insurance to federal employees, retirees, and their dependents. FEHBP is the country's largest employer-sponsored health insurance program; in 2010 the federal government spent $28.5 billion on FEHBP premiums for its nearly 8 million enrollees.[1]

Participation in FEHBP is voluntary. Enrollees can elect coverage in an approved plan for either individual or family coverage. FEHBP offers enrollees choices among a variety of different plans offered by private insurers. Enrollees can choose among nationally available fee-for-service plans and locally available plans. Many plans in FEHBP offer a choice between a standard option, a high option, and/or a high-deductible plan. The number of plans available to an enrollee varies according to where the enrollee resides, but most enrollees typically have a choice among 6 to 15 different plans. Premiums and cost-sharing requirements vary according to plan, and both the federal government and the enrollee contribute to the cost of premiums.

Prior to the creation of FEHBP in 1959, federal employees were not able to obtain health insurance through the federal government; instead, federal employees who wanted health insurance could voluntarily purchase coverage on their own or through the few union and employee association plans that offered plans to federal employees.[2] By 1950, it was common for employers in the private sector in the United States to offer health insurance and pay at least a portion of their employees' health insurance premiums. As early as 1951, it was recommended that the federal government begin following this practice.[3] After debate on whether and how the government should pursue this option, Congress passed the Federal Employees Health Benefits Act of 1959 (FEHBA, P.L. 86-382).[4]

FEHBA generally established parameters for eligibility; election of coverage; the types of health plans and benefits that may be offered; the level of the government's share of premiums; the establishment of an Employees Health Benefits Fund to pay for program expenses; and provisions for studies, reports, and audits. FEHBA also outlined the role of the Office of Personnel Management (OPM).[5] By law, OPM is given the authority to contract with insurers and to prescribe regulations to manage FEHBP, among other duties.[6]

FEHBA has been amended many times since its passage. The general model of FEHBP, consisting of enrollees choosing between multiple types of coverage offered by competing private insurers, has not changed. Employees and annuitants have always shared the cost of premiums

---

[1] Unpublished data from the Office of Personnel Management (OPM), based on March 2010 enrollment.

[2] U.S. Congress, House Committee on Post Office and Civil Service, *The Federal Employees Health Benefits Program: Possible Strategies for Reform*, committee print, prepared by Congressional Research Service, 101st Cong., 1st sess., May 24, 1989, Committee Print 101-5 (Washington: GPO, 1989).

[3] Odin W. Anderson and J. Joel May, *The Federal Employees Health Benefits Program, 1961-1968: A Model for National Health Insurance?* (Chicago: University of Chicago, 1971).

[4] Ibid.

[5] Until the passage of the Civil Service Reform Act of 1978 (P.L. 95-454), the Office of Personnel Management (OPM) was known as the Civil Service Commission. For the sake of clarity, in this report OPM is used even in the years prior to the change.

[6] For more information about OPM's authority within FEHBP, see CRS Report RS21974, *Federal Employees Health Benefits Program: Available Health Insurance Options*, by Annie L. Mach.

with the federal government, and employees and annuitants have generally always had access to the same plans at the same cost.[7]

However, many other aspects of FEHBP have been modified. For example, the determination of the government's share of premiums has changed several times, and the government's share of premiums has generally increased. In addition, eligibility, services, and benefits have generally been expanded in a number of ways. Congress, in its legislative authority, often has some part in modifying FEHBP, either in proposing changes to FEHBP or reacting to proposed changes.

Interest in FEHBP

Since its inception, policymakers and researchers have been interested in FEHBP both as a model for private and public health insurance programs (e.g., Medicare) and as an avenue for expanding coverage to certain individuals (e.g., the uninsured).[8] The FEHBP model consists of competing insurers providing numerous types of coverage to enrollees with minimal intervention from OPM. Many view this model as generally successful in giving enrollees the opportunity to make cost-conscious choices and in constraining the program's overall cost growth.

For this reason, some would like to export aspects of the FEHBP model to other health care programs. For example, some policymakers and researchers believe that Medicare could benefit from implementing aspects of the FEHBP model.[9] Others are interested in expanding access to FEHBP or creating new programs modeled after FEHBP to provide coverage to individuals who are not federal workers or annuitants, such as small business employees or the uninsured.[10] Some policymakers have embraced these ideas, introducing legislation to create new programs or opening FEHBP to individuals who are not federal employees or annuitants.[11] In the past, it has

---

[7] Certain plans offered in FEHBP are available only to certain types of employees and annuitants. For example, the Foreign Service Benefit Plan is available only to employees and annuitants who are American Foreign Service personnel. Non-postal employees and all annuitants pay the same premium for plans; however, postal employees have collective bargaining rights, and historically, the Postal Service's contribution to premiums for postal employees has been higher than for all other employees and annuitants.

[8] For examples of the various policymakers, including Members of Congress, Presidents, and presidential candidates, who have expressed interest in FEHBP as a model for other programs or in expanding access to FEHBP, see the following discussions: Walton Francis, *Putting Medicare Consumers in Charge* (Washington D.C.: The AEI Press, 2009), pp. 3-6; Beth C. Fuchs, *Increasing Health Insurance Coverage Through An Extended Federal Employees Health Benefits Program*, The Commonwealth Fund, December 2000, pp. 6-8, http://www.commonwealthfund.org/usr_doc/fuchs2_workable_414.pdf.

[9] The extent of support among policymakers and researchers for exporting FEHBP concepts to Medicare varies. For example, see Stuart M. Butler and Robert E. Moffit, "The FEHBP As A Model for A New Medicare Program," *Health Affairs*, vol. 14, no. 4 (Winter 1995); Karen Davis, Barbara S. Cooper, and Rose Capasso, *The Federal Employee Health Benefits Program: A Model for Workers, Not Medicare*, The Commonwealth Fund, November 2003; Roger Feldman, Kenneth E. Thorpe, and Bradley Gray, "The Federal Employees Health Benefits Plan," *Journal of Economic Perspectives*, vol. 16, no. 2 (Spring 2002); Walton Francis, *Putting Medicare Consumers in Charge* (Washington D.C.: The AEI Press, 2009); Mark Merlis, *The Federal Employees Health Benefits Program: Program Design, Recent Performance, and Implications for Medicare Reform*, Kaiser Family Foundation, May 2003.

[10] Stan Dorn and Jack A. Meyer, *Nine Billion Dollars a Year to Cover the Uninsured: Possible Common Ground for Significant, Incremental Process*, Economic and Social Research Institute, October 2002, http://www.esresearch.org/newsletter/october/summary4.htm; Beth C. Fuchs, *Increasing Health Insurance Coverage Through An Extended Federal Employees Health Benefits Program*, The Commonwealth Fund, December 2000, pp. 6-8, http://www.commonwealthfund.org/usr_doc/fuchs2_workable_414.pdf.

[11] For example, in the 112th Congress legislation has been introduced to enroll Medicare beneficiaries in FEHBP and to sunset the Medicare program (S. 2196) and also to open up FEHBP to individuals who are not federal employees or (continued...)

also been suggested that certain features of FEHBP are a good model for state-level health insurance exchanges,[12] and some would say that lessons learned from FEHBP may be instructive for state and federal officials that are establishing health benefit exchanges as created by the Patient Protection and Affordable Care Act (ACA, P.L. 111-148, as amended).[13]

Congressional interest in FEHBP often extends beyond FEHBP's potential applicability as a model for other health care programs or as an avenue to provide coverage. Congressional policymakers have some responsibility for FEHBP's viability and sustainability. Congress has a financial interest in the program, as the federal government has always paid a portion of FEHBP's costs. In addition, Congress has the legislative authority to restructure FEHBP to maintain or improve its function.[14]

Scope of Report

The purpose of the report is to provide information that helps explain how FEHBP has evolved into the program it is today and to understand how Congress has interacted with FEHBP in the past. The report includes short discussions of certain changes to the program. The report discusses how Congress has conditioned the use of federal funds on policy changes being implemented in FEHBP (**Table 1**); changed the formula for determining the government's share of FEHBP premiums (**Table 2**); modified eligibility for the program (**Table 3**); and implemented policies that affect the relationship between Medicare and FEHBP (**Table 4**).

In addition, the **Appendix** contains a summary of the enacting FEHBP legislation and summaries of selected laws that have since amended or otherwise affected FEHBP. The summaries are presented in chronological order. The summaries in the **Appendix** provide more detailed examination of the legislation discussed in the body of this report, as well as summaries of additional legislation that affects FEHBP.

(...continued)
annuitants (H.R. 429).

[12] See, for example, Robert E. Moffit, *State-Based Health Reform: A Comparison of Health Insurance Exchanges and the Federal Employees Health Benefits Program*, The Heritage Foundation, No. 1515, June 20, 2007, http://hss.state.ak.us/hspc/files/200710_state_fedbenefit.pdf.

[13] Timothy D. McBride, Abigail R. Barker, Lisa M. Pollack, et al., "Federal Employees Health Program Experiences Lack of Competition in Some Areas, Raising Cost Concerns for Exchange Plans," *Health Affairs*, vol. 31, no. 6 (June 2012), pp. 1321-1328.

[14] Also, as federal employees, Members of Congress and congressional staff are currently eligible to participate in FEHBP; however, ACA includes a provision that will affect whether Members and certain congressional staff can access FEHBP. For more information about health benefits for Members of Congress and changes under ACA, see CRS Report RS21982, *Health Benefits for Members of Congress*, by Ada S. Cornell.

> **Information Not Included in This Report**
>
> This report includes summaries of laws or provisions of laws that have directly amended or otherwise caused policy changes to FEHBP. The report does not summarize any laws or provisions of laws that may apply generally, rather than specifically, to FEHBP. For example, the Health Insurance Portability and Accountability Act of 1996 (HIPAA, P.L. 104-191) includes provisions that apply generally to group health plans. While plans provided under FEHBP are presumed to fall under the definition of "group health plan," and OPM requires FEHBP plans to comply with HIPAA provisions, HIPAA does not specifically apply to FEHBP, and it is not summarized in this report.
>
> In addition, this report does not cover any changes made to FEHBP by OPM. Statute gives OPM broad authority to administer FEHBP, and in exercising that authority, OPM can implement changes to FEHBP.[15] For example, OPM issues "call letters" to FEHBP plans each year, which outline its policy goals for the upcoming year. In the call letter for the 1990 contract year, OPM used its authority to require all plans to include coverage of prescription drugs.[16] Subsequent call letters have expanded and modified OPM's prescription drug requirements. In another example, OPM recently published an interim final rule that extends FEHBP eligibility to temporary federal firefighters.[17] OPM has indicated that doing so was within its authority to include or exclude employees in FEHBP.[18]
>
> Finally, this report does not summarize any laws or provisions of laws that provide technical clarifications, non-substantive grammatical changes, or name changes to FEHBP.

Conditions on FEHBP Use of Federal Funds

Congress can place conditions on the use of federal funds, and it has done so to effect and maintain policy changes in FEHBP. For example, in 1983 Congress passed a law that prohibited using appropriated federal funds to cover abortions, except when the life of the woman was in danger.[19] This provision was renewed with few changes every year except 1994 and 1995, when the 103rd Congress excluded the provision.[20] The reinstated provision prohibited the use of funds except when the life of the woman was in danger or in cases of rape or incest; this provision has been included in subsequent appropriations bills each year (as of the date of this report).[21]

Table 1 summarizes provisions in several laws that enact policy changes in FEHBP by conditioning the use of federal funds.

---

[15] In at least one instance, Congress has acted to block implementation of a policy change to FEHBP that was created by OPM, in its authority to administer FEHBP. See P.L. 102-393 in the **Appendix** for more details.

[16] FEHB Program Carrier Letter, March 30, 1989.

[17] 77 *Federal Register* 42417, July 17, 2012.

[18] Letter from John Berry, Director of the Office of Personnel Management, to The Honorable Tom Coburn, Senator, August 3, 2012.

[19] This legislative restriction on FEHBP funds followed an earlier administrative attempt by OPM to eliminate non-life-saving abortion coverage. OPM's actions were challenged by federal employee unions, and a federal district court later concluded that the agency acted outside the scope of its authority. In American Federation of Government Employees v. AFL-CIO, 525 F.Supp. 250 (1981), the court found that absent a specific congressional statutory directive, there was no basis for OPM's actions.

[20] **Table 1** and the **Appendix** only include descriptions of laws that introduced this provision or failed to include it.

[21] For further analysis of legislation related to coverage for abortion, see CRS Report RL33467, *Abortion: Judicial History and Legislative Response*, by Jon O. Shimabukuro.

Table 1. Provisions of Laws Conditioning the Use of Federal Funds for FEHBP

Year	Authorizing Statute	Change in How Federal Funds May Be Used in FEHBP
1983	A Joint Resolution Making Further Continuing Appropriations for the Fiscal Year 1984 (P.L. 98-151)	Restricted use of funds to pay for abortions or administrative expenses for any FEHBP plan that provides benefits or coverage for abortions, except when the life of the woman is in danger
		Provision has been applied to FEHBP every year except 1994 and 1995; since 1996 the provision has included an exception for cases of rape and incest
1993	Treasury, Postal Service, and General Government Appropriations Act, 1993 (P.L. 102-393)	Prohibited use of funds appropriated by the Act to implement changes proposed by OPM that would affect Medicare beneficiaries
1997	Assisted Suicide Funding Restriction Act of 1997 (P.L. 105-12)	Prohibited use of federal funds for benefits and services related to assisted suicide and prohibits OPM from contracting with plans that include coverage for these benefits and services
1999	Omnibus Consolidated and Emergency Supplemental Appropriations Act, 1999 (P.L. 105-277)	Required all FEHBP plans to cover contraceptives, with the exception of certain plans that object to such coverage on the basis of religious beliefs
		Provision has been applied to FEHBP every year since 1999

Source: CRS analysis of selected legislation.

Premium Determinations

Over the years, the determination of the government's share of premiums has changed, and the percentage of the government's share of premiums has increased overall. In the enacting legislation, the government's share was set at 50% of the premium, and it had to fall within a specified dollar range. The determination changed little until 1971, when the "big six" formula was created. The formula was equal to the simple average of the premiums of six health plans offered in FEHBP that met the criteria specified in statute. The government's share was originally set at 40% of the simple average of the big six premiums and increased to 50% in 1974.

The big six formula was in place with few changes until 1997. The passage of the Balanced Budget Act of 1997 (P.L. 105-33) introduced the formula for determining the government's share of premiums that is in effect today. The government contributes 72% of the weighted average premium of all plans, not to exceed 75% of the premium for any one plan (calculated separately for individual and family coverage).

Table 2. Provisions of Laws Related to Changes in How the Government's Share of the Premium Is Determined

Passed	Authorizing Statute	Change in How the Government's Share of the Premium is Determined
1959	The Federal Employees Health Benefits Act of 1959 (P.L. 86-382)	Set the government's share of premiums at 50% of the lowest rate charged by a carrier, and required the government's share to fall in a specified dollar range. The dollar range was different depending on plan type (individual or family) and the enrollee's gender and family situation
1964	To Amend the Federal Employees Health Benefits Act of 1959 to Remove Certain Inequities in the Application of Such Act, to Improve the Administration Thereof, and for Other Purposes (P.L. 88-284)	Made the government's share of premiums the same for *all* enrollees according to plan type (individual or family), regardless of gender and family situation
1966	The Federal Salary and Fringe Benefits Act of 1966 (P.L. 89-504)	Changed the government's share of premiums from falling in a specified dollar range to a fixed-dollar amount
1970	An Act to Increase the Contribution by the Federal Government to the Cost of Health Benefits Insurance, and for Other Purposes (P.L. 91-418)	Altered the determination of the government's share of premiums by creating the "big six" formula, calculated separately for individual and family plans Set the government's share at 40% of the simple average of the big six premiums
1974	An Act to Increase the Contribution of the Government to the Costs of Health Benefits for Federal Employees, and for Other Purposes (P.L. 93-246)	Increased the government's share of the FEHBP plan premium from 40% to 50% of the simple average of the big six premiums Set the maximum government share at 75% of the total premium for any one plan
1989	Relating to the Method by Which Government Contributions to the Federal Employees Health Benefits Program Shall be Computed for 1990 or 1991 if no Government-Wide Indemnity Benefit Plan Participates in that Year (P.L. 101-76)	Adjusted the big six formula to account for the absence of one of the plan types specified in the formula
1990	Omnibus Budget Reconciliation Act of 1990 (P.L. 101-508)	Extended the restructured big six formula for calculating the government's share of premiums through 1993
1993	Omnibus Budget Reconciliation Act of 1993 (P.L. 103-66)	Extended the restructured big six formula for calculating the government's share of premiums through 1998 (with modifications for contract years 1997 and 1998)
1997	Balanced Budget Act of 1997 (P.L. 105-33)	Modified the formula for determining the government's share of premiums by requiring that OPM determine the weighted average premium of all plans in FEHBP each year, calculated separately for individual and family plans Required that the biweekly government share of a premium is equal to 72% of this average, not to exceed 75% of any given plan's premium

Source: CRS analysis of selected legislation.

Eligibility

FEHBP-eligible participants specified in the enacting legislation included current federal employees and annuitants who retired *after* July 1, 1960.[22] Family members of employees and annuitants were also eligible. See the text box, "Eligibility Under the Federal Employees Health Benefits Act (P.L. 86-382)," for a complete list of eligibility under the enacting legislation. Since the enactment of FEHBA, eligibility to enroll in FEHBP has generally been extended to more categories of federal employees, annuitants, and their family and ex-family members.

> **Eligibility Under the Federal Employees Health Benefits Act (P.L. 86-382)**
>
> Specifically, the enacting legislation provided that the following individuals were eligible for FEHBP: (1) any appointed or elected officer or employee in the executive, judicial, or legislative branch of the federal government, including a government-owned or controlled corporation (except any corporation under the supervision of the Farm Credit Administration); (2) any appointed or elected officer or employee of the municipal government of the District of Columbia; (3) employees of Gallaudet College; (4) annuitants who retire on an immediate annuity after 12 or more years of service or for a disability and were enrolled in a FEHBP plan for at least five years immediately prior to retirement, or enrolled from the earliest opportunity to do so; (5) a member of a family who receives an immediate annuity as the survivor of an annuitant or employee who dies after completing five or more years of service; (6) an employee who receives monthly compensation under the Federal Employees' Compensation Act (FECA, P.L. 64-267) as a result of a work-related injury or illness, and who is determined by the Secretary of Labor to be unable to return to duty; (7) a member of a family who receives monthly compensation under FECA as the surviving beneficiary of an employee who has sustained work-related injuries or illnesses; (8) an employee's or annuitant's spouse; (9) an employee's or annuitant's unmarried child under the age of 19 years, including an adopted child, a stepchild, and a recognized natural child who lives with the employee or annuitant in a regular parent-child relationship; (10) an employee's or annuitant's unmarried child who, regardless of age, is incapable of self-support because of mental or physical incapacity that existed prior to the child reaching the age of 19 years.

FEHBP has also been expanded in that in 1978 it was extended to part-time employees, and in 1988 it was extended to certain temporary workers. In 1988, Congress also authorized temporary continuation of coverage (TCC), whereby employees separated from service for reasons other than gross misconduct can continue coverage in FEHBP.[23] TCC enrollees must pay the entire FEHBP premium, both the employer's and the employees' share, as well as a 2% administrative fee. In general, TCC is available to separating employees and their dependents for up to 18 months after the date of separation; however, there are exceptions, such as 36 months of available coverage for children aging out of their parent's plans. TCC coverage has been modified for certain employees and dependents since originally enacted.

---

[22] In 1960, Congress passed The Retired Federal Employees Health Benefits Act (P.L. 86-724), which authorized the creation of a health benefits program for federal employees who retired or became disabled *before* July 1, 1960, and their family members. The program, "retired FEHBP," was patterned after the existing FEHBP. In 1974, Congress passed An Act to Increase the Contribution of the Government to the Costs of Health Benefits for Federal Employees, and for Other Purposes (P.L. 93-246), which allowed annuitants participating or eligible to participate in retired FEHBP and their family members to participate in regular FEHBP. This report does not include summaries of legislation or provisions of legislation that affect only retired FEHBP.

[23] TCC mirrors coverage created under Title X of the Consolidated Omnibus Budget Reconciliation Act of 1985 (COBRA; P.L. 99-272), which provides similar protections for private sector employees. For more information about COBRA, see CRS Report R40142, *Health Insurance Continuation Coverage Under COBRA*, by Janet Kinzer.

Table 3. Laws Affecting Eligibility for FEHBP

	Authorizing Statute	Change in Eligibility for FEHBP
1959	The Federal Employees Health Benefits Act of 1959 (P.L. 86-382)	Authorized coverage for federal employees, annuitants who retired after July 1, 1960,[a] dependents of employees and annuitants, as well as other specified individuals[b]
1960	The Postal Employees Salary Increase Act of 1960 (P.L. 86-568)	Authorized coverage for Agriculture Stabilization and Conservation County Committee employees and their dependents
1964	To Amend the Federal Employees Health Benefits Act of 1959 to Remove Certain Inequities in the Application of Such Act, to Improve the Administration Thereof, and for Other Purposes (P.L. 88-284)	Authorized coverage for employees receiving compensation because of work-related injury, foster children, and unmarried children up to age 21
1964	To Amend the Federal Employees Health Benefits Act of 1959 and the Federal Employees Group Life Insurance Act of 1954 (P.L. 88-531)	Authorized coverage for certain United States Commissioners and their dependents
1964	To Amend the Federal Employees Health Benefits Act of 1959 and the Federal Employees Group Life Insurance Act of 1954 (P.L. 88-631)	Authorized coverage for teachers in D.C. who had been temporarily employed as teachers for a total of at least two years
1966	To Preserve the Benefits of the Civil Service Retirement Act, the Federal Employees Group Life Insurance Act of 1954, and the Federal Employees Health Benefits Act of 1959 for Congressional Employees Receiving Certain Congressional Staff Fellowships (P.L. 89-379)	Authorized coverage for congressional staff receiving certain congressional staff fellowships
1966	The Federal Salary and Fringe Benefits Act of 1966 (P.L. 89-504)	Authorized coverage for dependent children from age 21 to 22 Permitted certain employees on leave without pay to continue or acquire coverage
1968	The National Guard Technicians Act of 1968 (P.L. 90-486)	Authorized coverage for National Guard technicians and their dependents
1968	The Federal Magistrates Act (P.L. 90-578)	Authorized coverage for United States magistrates, their clerical and secretarial assistants, and their dependents
1969	The Foreign Assistance Act of 1969 (P.L. 91-175)	Authorized coverage for employees during a period of transfer to employment with an international organization
1970	An Act to Increase the Contribution by the Federal Government to the Cost of Health Benefits Insurance, and for Other Purposes (P.L. 91-418)	Authorized coverage for: (1) family members who received an immediate annuity as the survivor of an employee or of a retired employee in the event that the deceased had completed less than five years of creditable service; (2) noncitizen employees whose permanent duty station is in the Panama Canal Zone
1971	The Intergovernmental Personnel Act of 1970 (P.L. 91-648)	Authorized coverage for federal employees assigned to state or local governments Authorized coverage for state or local government employees who were assigned to an executive agency in the federal government
1973	To Extend Civil Service Federal Employees Group Life Insurance and Federal Employees Health Benefits Coverage to United States Nationals Employed by the Federal Government (P.L. 93-160)	Authorized coverage for otherwise eligible United States nationals employed at permanent duty stations outside the United States and the Panama Canal Zone

	Authorizing Statute	Change in Eligibility for FEHBP
1976	To Amend Title 5, United States Code, to Restore Eligibility for Health Benefits Coverage to Certain Individuals Whose Survivor Annuities are Restored (P.L. 94-342)	Authorized coverage for a surviving spouse when the survivor annuity was terminated because of remarriage to re-enroll in FEHBP if the survivor annuity is restored
1978	The Federal Employees Part Time Career Employment Act of 1978 (P.L. 95-437)	Authorized coverage for part-time career employees and their dependents
1978	To Amend Subchapter m of Chapter 83 of Title 5, United States Code, to Provide that Employees who Retire After 5 Years of Service, in Certain Instances, May be Eligible to Retain their Life and Health Insurance Benefits, and for Other Purposes (P.L. 95-583)	Reduced the length of creditable service required by a retiring employee in order to retain FEHBP coverage into retirement from 12 years to 5 years
1979	To Make Certain Technical and Clerical Amendments to Title 5, United States Code (P.L. 96-54)	Redefined "employee" for the purpose of FEHBP coverage to exclude the previous reference to United States Commissioners
1979	The Panama Canal Act of 1979 (P.L. 96-70)	Excluded individuals from FEHBP who were not citizens or nationals of the United States, and whose permanent duty station was outside the United States, *unless* the individual was an employee on September 30, 1979, by reason of service in specified government agencies
1980	To Amend Provisions of Chapters 83 and 89 of Title 5, United States Code, Which Relate to Survivor Benefits for Certain Dependent Children, and for Other Purposes (P.L. 96-179)	Eliminated the "lives with" requirement for a natural child to be covered by FEHBP and added a dependency requirement for all children
1984	The Civil Service Retirement Spouse Equity Act of 1984 (P.L. 98-615)	Authorized coverage for former spouses of employed, retired, or separated federal employees
1985	An Act to Provide that Employee Organizations Ineligible to Participate in the FEHBP Solely Because Applications for Approval Must be Filed Before January 1, 1980, May Apply to Become so Eligible, and For Other Purposes (P.L. 99-53)	Permitted certain disability annuitants who were later restored to federal employment to enroll in a FEHBP plan if the annuitant had been enrolled in any such plan immediately prior to termination of employment
1986	The Federal Employees Benefits Improvement Act of 1986 (P.L. 99-251)	Gave OPM the authority to waive the five years of service requirement for individuals to have FEHBP coverage in retirement in cases of exceptional circumstances
1986	The Federal Employees' Retirement System Act of 1986 (P.L. 99-335)	Authorized coverage for individuals first employed by the District of Columbia government before October 1, 1987
1986	The Intelligence Authorization Act for Fiscal Year 1987 (P.L. 99-569)	Authorized coverage for certain former spouses of Central Intelligence Agency (CIA) employees
1987	The Foreign Relations Authorization Act, Fiscal Years 1988 and 1989 (P.L. 100-204)	Authorized coverage for certain former spouses of employees or former employees of the Foreign Service
1988	The Federal Employees' Retirement System Technical Corrections Act (P.L. 100-238)	Declared that certain nonfederal employees eligible for FEHBP benefits are no longer entitled to such benefits after October 1, 1988
1988	Federal Employees Health Benefits Amendments Act of 1988 (P.L. 100-654)	Created temporary continuation of coverage (TCC) in FEHBP whereby federal employees separated from service and certain dependents can maintain FEHBP
		Directed OPM to prescribe regulations offering FEHBP to certain temporary federal employees

	Authorizing Statute	**Change in Eligibility for FEHBP**
1988	Office of Federal Procurement Policy Act Amendments of 1988 (P.L. 100-679)	Authorized coverage for certain individuals employed by former Presidents and Vice Presidents
1990	Foreign Relations Authorization Act, Fiscal Years 1990 and 1991 (P.L. 101-246)	Authorized coverage for former spouses of certain former Foreign Service employees in certain circumstances
1990	Foreign Operations, Export Financing, and Related Programs Appropriations (P.L. 101-513)	Authorized coverage for U.S. hostages in Iraq, Kuwait, and those captured in Lebanon, and their family members, while they remained in hostage status and for 12 months thereafter
1990	Elimination of Post-1968 Service Prerequisite for Retirement Credit and Other Benefits (P.L. 101-530)	Provided that post-1968 service by National Guard technicians is not a required prerequisite for entitlement to FEHBP
1991	Intelligence Authorization Act, Fiscal Year 1991 (P.L. 102-88)	Provided that a former spouse of a CIA employee who is not eligible to enroll or continue enrollment in a FEHBP plan solely because of remarriage before age 55 may enroll in a FEHBP plan under certain circumstances
1991	Legislative Branch Appropriations Act, 1992 (P.L. 102-90)	Authorized coverage for employees of the Senate Employee Child Care Center
1992	National Defense Authorization Act for Fiscal Year 1993 (P.L. 102-484)	Provided for special rules with regard to TCC under FEHBP if the basis for TCC is involuntary separation from a position in or under the Department of Defense due to a reduction in force
1994	FEGLI Living Benefits Act, 1994 (P.L. 103-409)	Authorized coverage for employees of the Office of the Comptroller of the Currency and the Office of Thrift Supervision whose health coverage, provided under their organizations' plans, terminates
1996	National Defense Authorization Act for Fiscal Year 1996 (P.L. 104-106)	Allowed individuals who separate from certain positions in or under the Department of Defense or the Department of Energy, to continue coverage under FEHBP and be liable for no more than the employee's share of FEHBP premiums
1996	Omnibus Consolidated Appropriations Act, 1997 (P.L. 104-208)	Required OPM to prescribe regulations under which surviving children, whose survivor annuity was terminated because of marriage and is later restored (because the marriage ends), may enroll in a FEHBP plan
1998	Federal Employees Health Care Protection Act of 1998 (P.L. 105-266)	Authorized coverage for employees of the Federal Deposit Insurance Corporation and the Board of Governors of the Federal Reserve Board whose health coverage, provided under their organizations' plans, terminates
1998	District of Columbia Courts and Justice Technical Corrections Act of 1998 (P.L. 105-274)	Authorized coverage for District of Columbia public defender service employees
2000	Federal Employees Health Benefits Children's Equity Act of 2000 (P.L. 106-394)	Mandated that federal employees legally required to provide health insurance coverage to a dependent child do so under FEHBP, if the child does not otherwise have coverage
2000	District of Columbia Appropriations Act, 2001 (P.L. 106-522)	Authorized coverage for certain employees of the District of Columbia
2002	To Amend Title 5, United States Code, to Allow Certain Catch-up Contributions to the Thrift Savings Plan to be Made by Participants Age 50 or Over (P.L. 107-304)	Authorized coverage for employees of the Overseas Private Investment Corporation (OPIC) when OPIC-administered plans terminate

Laws Affecting the Federal Employees Health Benefits Program (FEHBP)

	Authorizing Statute	Change in Eligibility for FEHBP
2002	Bob Stump National Defense Authorization Act for Fiscal Year 2003 (P.L. 107-314)	Extended the ability of individuals who are involuntarily separated from military service, or voluntarily separated from a surplus position in the Departments of Defense or Energy due to a reduction in force, to continue coverage under FEHBP
2004	State Justice Institute Reauthorization Act of 2004 (P.L. 108-372)	Authorized coverage for State Justice Institute employees who commenced employment on or after October 1, 1988
2004	Ronald W. Reagan National Defense Authorization Act for Fiscal Year 2005 (P.L. 108-375)	Provided for special rules for TCC under FEHBP for certain federal employees
2007	A bill to amend chapter 89 of title 5, United States Code, to make individuals employed by the Roosevelt Campobello International Park Commission eligible to obtain Federal health insurance (P.L. 110-74)	Authorized coverage for U.S. citizens employed by the Roosevelt Campobello International Park Commission
2008	A bill to provide for certain Federal employee benefits to be continued for certain employees of the Senate Restaurants after operations of the Senate Restaurants are contracted to be performed by a private business concern, and for other purposes (P.L. 110-279)	Permitted specified Senate Restaurants employees working under the Architect of the Capitol to elect to continue coverage under FEHBP after operations of the Senate Restaurants are contracted out
2008	National Aeronautics and Space Administration (NASA) Authorization Act of 2008 (P.L. 110-422)	Provided for special rules for TCC under FEHBP for employees who are terminated or separated from certain positions at NASA
2010	Patient Protection and Affordable Care Act of 2010 (P.L. 111-148, as amended)	Made a requirement that Members of Congress and certain congressional staff, in relation to their federal employment, may *only* enroll in health plans created under ACA, or offered through a health insurance exchange, instead of FEHBP
		Allowed all adult children (including married children) up to age 26 to remain/enroll on their parent's FEHBP plan
		Allowed certain Indian tribes and organizations to purchase FEHBP for tribal employees[c]

Source: CRS analysis of selected legislation.

a. In 1960, Congress passed The Retired Federal Employees Health Benefits Act (P.L. 86-724), which authorized the creation of a health benefits program for federal employees who retired or became disabled *before* July 1, 1960, and their family members. The program, "retired FEHBP," was patterned after the existing FEHBP. In 1974, Congress passed An Act to Increase the Contribution of the Government to the Costs of Health benefits for Federal Employees, and for Other Purposes (P.L. 93-246), which allowed annuitants participating or eligible to participate in retired FEHBP and their family members to participate in regular FEHBP. This report does not include summaries of legislation or provisions of legislation that only affect retired FEHBP.

b. For a detailed list of individuals eligible for FEHBP under the enacting legislation, see the text box "Eligibility Under the Federal Employees Health Benefits Act (P.L. 86-382)."

c. This provision was included in the Indian Health Care Improvement Reauthorization and Extension Act of 2009 (S. 1790), which was enacted by §10221(a) of the Patient Protection and Affordable Care Act of 2010 (P.L. 111-148).

Medicare and FEHBP

FEHBP was established five years prior to Medicare, and in the early years there was little interaction between the programs. This was largely because, in general, federal employees and annuitants were not eligible for Medicare based on their federal employment. This changed in 1982 when Congress passed the Tax Equity and Fiscal Responsibility Act (P.L. 97-248), which applied Medicare's hospital insurance tax to federal employment, thereby enabling federal workers to be eligible for Medicare based on their federal employment.[24]

Table 4. Provisions Related to Changing How FEHBP and Medicare Interact

Passed	Authorizing Statute	Change in Medicare-FEHBP Relationship
1982	The Tax Equity and Fiscal Responsibility Act of 1982 (P.L. 97-248)	Applied Medicare's Hospital Insurance tax to federal employment
		Provided that Medicare payments are secondary for services provided to federal employees and their spouses aged 65 to 69 if covered under FEHBP. This provision did not apply to federal annuitants; Medicare remained the primary payer for annuitants
1986	The Consolidated Omnibus Budget Reconciliation Act of 1985 (P.L. 99-272)	Provided that Medicare payments are secondary for services provided to federal employees (i.e., workers) and their spouses aged 65 and older if covered under FEHBP
		This provision did not apply to federal annuitants; Medicare remained the primary payer for annuitants
1988	Medicare Catastrophic Coverage Act of 1988 (P.L. 100-360)	This Act was repealed,[a] but had it not been repealed, it would have required OPM to reduce the FEHBP premiums charged to Medicare-eligible retirees who are also participating in FEHBP
1990	Omnibus Budget Reconciliation Act of 1990 (P.L. 101-508)	Required improved coordination between Medicare and FEHBP
		Applied certain Medicare Part A payment limits to services provided to retired FEHBP enrollees aged 65 and over *who are not* covered by Medicare Part A[b]
1992	Treasury, Postal Service, and General Government Appropriations Act (P.L. 102-393)	Prohibited the use of funds appropriated by the Act to implement changes proposed by OPM that would affect Medicare beneficiaries
1993	Omnibus Budget Reconciliation Act of 1993 (P.L. 103-66)	Applied certain Medicare Part B payment limits to services provided to retired FEHBP enrollees aged 65 and older *who do not* participate in Medicare Part B[b]

Source: CRS analysis of selected legislation.

a. The law was repealed by the Medicare Catastrophic Coverage Repeal Act of 1989 (P.L. 101-234).

b. Medicare has specific rules for payment of covered benefits, and all Medicare beneficiaries, including those who also have coverage under FEHBP, are subject to those rules. For more information on the rules, see CRS Report RL30526, *Medicare Payment Policies*, coordinated by Paulette C. Morgan.

---

[24] While federal employment did not count toward Medicare eligibility prior to 1982, federal employees who were employed in the private sector at one time and were subject to Medicare's hospital insurance tax could have been eligible for Medicare based on their prior private sector employment.

Appendix. FEHBP Legislative History

The Federal Employees Health Benefits Act of 1959 (P.L. 86-382), September 28, 1959

Effective July 1, 1960, the Act authorized the creation of the Federal Employees Health Benefits program (FEHBP) for the federal workforce. The Act established the general parameters for program operation, which included detailing eligibility and enrollment procedures; describing the types of benefits that may be provided; determining the level of government's share of premiums; and outlining the role of the Office of Personnel Management (OPM).[25]

FEHBP-eligible participants specified in the enacting legislation included current federal employees, and annuitants who retired *after* July 1, 1960, either on an immediate annuity with at least 12 years of service or for a disability.[26] Annuitants were also required either to be enrolled in a FEHBP plan for at least five years immediately prior to retirement, or enrolled from the earliest opportunity to do so. Family members of employees and annuitants were also eligible.[27]

OPM was allowed to contract or approve the following types of health benefit plans to participate in FEHBP:[28]

- Service Benefit Plan—one government-wide plan (offering two levels of benefits) under which payment is made by an insurer under contracts with providers for the benefits described.

- Indemnity Benefit Plan—one government-wide plan (offering two levels of benefits) under which an insurer agrees to pay certain sums of money for the benefits described.[29]

- Employee Organization Plans—plans providing health benefits to members of the organization as of July 1, 1959, that are sponsored or underwritten, and administered, in whole or part, by employee organizations, and are available only to employees and annuitants (and members of their families) who at the time of enrollment are members of the organization.

---

[25] Prior to the enactment of the Civil Service Reform Act of 1978 (P.L. 95-454), the Office of Personnel Management (OPM) was called the Civil Service Commission. For the sake of clarity, this report only refers to "OPM," even when discussing legislation passed prior to the Civil Service Reform Act of 1978.

[26] In 1960, Congress passed The Retired Federal Employees Health Benefits Act (P.L. 86-724) which authorized the creation of a health benefits program for federal employees who retired or became disabled *before* July 1, 1960, and their family members. The program, "retired FEHBP," was patterned after the existing FEHBP. In 1974, Congress passed An Act to Increase the Contribution of the Government to the Costs of Health benefits for Federal Employees, and for Other Purposes (P.L. 93-246), which allowed annuitants participating or eligible to participate in retired FEHBP and their family members to participate in regular FEHBP. This report does not include summaries of legislation or provisions of legislation that only affect retired FEHBP.

[27] See the text box, "Eligibility Under the Federal Employees Health Benefits Act (P.L. 86-382)," for a detailed list of individuals eligible for FEHBP under the enacting legislation.

[28] §4 of P.L. 86-382.

[29] According to OPM, a major difference between the Service Benefit Plan and the Indemnity Benefit Plan is that the Service Benefit Plan pays providers directly for health care services, while enrollees in the Indemnity Benefit Plan pay the provider and the Plan reimburses the enrollee.

- Comprehensive Medical Plans—either *group-practice prepayment plans* which offer benefits on a prepaid basis provided by physicians practicing as a group in a common center or centers, or *individual-practice prepayment plans* which offer health services on a prepaid basis provided by individual physicians who agree to accept the payments provided by the plans as full payment for covered services rendered by them.

The government's share of premiums in FEHBP plans was dependent on the type of plan and the type of enrollee.[30]

- For the service benefit plan and the indemnity plan, the government's share was 50% of the lowest rate charged by a carrier, and
  - for an employee or annuitant with individual coverage, the biweekly government share could not be less than $1.25 and not more than $1.75;
  - for an employee or annuitant with family coverage, the biweekly government share could not be less than $3.00 and not more than $4.25;
  - for a female employee or annuitant with a nondependent husband with family coverage, the biweekly government share could not be less than $1.75 and not more than $2.50.
- For employees and annuitants enrolled in either employee organization plans or comprehensive medical plans,
  - the government's share was 50% of the biweekly premium as long as the biweekly premium was less than $2.50 for individual coverage and less than $6.00 for family coverage;
  - for a female employee or annuitant who had a nondependent husband and family coverage, the government shared 30% of the premium (as long as the biweekly premium was less than $6.00).

The Postal Employees Salary Increase Act of 1960 (P.L. 86-568), July 1, 1960

The Act authorized FEHBP coverage for Agriculture Stabilization and Conservation County Committee employees and their dependents.[31]

To Amend the Federal Employees Health Benefits Act of 1959 to Provide Additional Choice of Health Benefits Plans, and for Other Purposes (P.L. 88-59), July 8, 1963

The Act extended the time period for acceptance of applications from qualified employee organizations wanting to participate in FEHBP from December 31, 1959 to January 1, 1964. The Act also eliminated the requirement for an employee organization to have offered health care benefits to its members prior to submitting an application for FEHBP. Prior to the passage of the

---

[30] §7 of P.L. 86-382.
[31] §115(d) of P.L. 86-568.

Act, for an employee organization to be approved to offer coverage under FEHBP, it had to have been providing its members with health care benefits by July 1, 1959 (see P.L. 86-382).

To Amend the Federal Employees Health Benefits Act of 1959 to Remove Certain Inequities in the Application of Such Act, to Improve the Administration Thereof, and for Other Purposes (P.L. 88-284), March 17, 1964

The Act broadened FEHBP coverage to include employees concurrently receiving compensation as the result of an on-the-job injury, foster children, and unmarried children up to age 21 (raised from age 19). The Act also eased the requirements for employees to continue their FEHBP coverage in retirement by allowing them to continue coverage if they were enrolled in a FEHBP plan by December 31, 1964.[32]

At the request of OPM, the Act also gave OPM discretionary authority to terminate FEHBP plan contracts with any carrier who did not enroll at least 300 employees and annuitants (excluding family members) during the preceding two contract terms. The Act made the government's share of the premium the same for all enrollees, regardless of gender.[33]

Finally, the Act changed the government's share of premiums for employee organization plans and comprehensive medical plans. For an employee or annuitant enrolled in one of these plans for which the biweekly premium was less than twice the government's share established for service benefit plans and indemnity plans, the government's share was 50% of the premium (for both individual and family plans).[34]

To Amend the Federal Employees Health Benefits Act of 1959 and the Federal Employees Group Life Insurance Act of 1954 (P.L. 88-531), August 31, 1964

The Act authorized FEHBP coverage for certain United States Commissioners to whom the Civil Service Retirement Act (P.L. 71-279) applies and their dependents.

To Amend the Federal Employees Health Benefits Act of 1959 and the Federal Employees Group Life Insurance Act of 1954 (P.L. 88-631), October 6, 1964

The Act authorized FEHBP coverage for teachers in the District of Columbia if they had been temporarily employed as teachers for a total of at least two years.

---

[32] Under FEHBP's enacting legislation (P.L. 86-382), the continuation of health benefits coverage into retirement required an annuitant to have had at least five years of FEHBP coverage immediately prior to retirement, or had to have been enrolled in FEHBP continuously from the first opportunity to enroll. Many employees had not realized the importance of enrolling at their first opportunity and, without P.L. 88-284, would have been ineligible to continue their FEHBP enrollment into retirement.

[33] FEHBP's enacting legislation (P.L. 86-382) provided for a smaller government contribution for women with nondependent husbands who were enrolled in a family plan.

[34] §7 of P.L. 88-284.

To Preserve the Benefits of the Civil Service Retirement Act, the Federal Employees Group Life Insurance Act of 1954, and the Federal Employees Health Benefits Act of 1959 for Congressional Employees Receiving Certain Congressional Staff Fellowships (P.L. 89-379), March 30, 1966

The Act extended FEHBP coverage to congressional employees receiving certain congressional staff fellowships.

The Federal Salary and Fringe Benefits Act of 1966 (P.L. 89-504), July 18, 1966

The Act amended FEHBP to change the fixed-dollar government share of the cost of plan premiums. The biweekly government share for *all* plan types for individual enrollment became $1.62; the biweekly government share for *all* plan types for family enrollment became $3.94. Neither could exceed 50% of the total premium.[35]

In addition, FEHBP coverage for dependent children was extended from age 21 to age 22,[36] and employees who were on leave without pay to serve as full-time officers or employees of employee organizations[37] were permitted to continue or acquire coverage.[38]

The National Guard Technicians Act of 1968 (P.L. 90-486), August 13, 1968

National Guard technicians were converted to federal employee status effective January 1, 1969, and the Act authorized FEHBP coverage for them and their dependents.[39]

The Federal Magistrates Act (P.L. 90-578), October 17, 1968

The Act authorized FEHBP coverage for United States magistrates, their clerical and secretarial assistants, and their dependents.[40]

The Foreign Assistance Act of 1969 (P.L. 91-175), December 30, 1969

The Act granted federal employees the option of continuing participation in FEHBP during a period of transfer to employment with an international organization.[41]

---

[35] §602 of P.L. 89-504.

[36] §601 of P.L. 89-504.

[37] An "employee organization" is defined in P.L. 86-382 as "an association or other organization of employees which is national in scope or in which membership is open to all employees of a government department, agency, or independent establishment who are eligible to enroll in a health benefits plan under this Act."

[38] §406 of P.L. 89-504.

[39] §3 of P.L. 90-486.

[40] §634 of P.L. 90-578.

[41] §502 of P.L. 91-175.

An Act to Increase the Contribution by the Federal Government to the Cost of Health Benefits Insurance, and for Other Purposes (P.L. 91-418), September 25, 1970

The Act altered the determination of the government's share of plan premiums in an effort to "provide automatic indexing of the government contribution to reflect increases in medical price inflation."[42]

Beginning with the first pay period in 1971, the Act established what is commonly referred to as the "big six" formula. The big six formula is equal to the simple average of the premiums calculated separately for individual and family coverage, (using the high option where a high and standard option are offered) of the two government-wide plans (the service benefit plan and the indemnity plan), and the two employee organization plans and the two comprehensive medical plans with the highest enrollment. The Act set the government's share at 40% of the simple average of the big six premiums.[43]

The Act permitted family members who received an immediate annuity as the survivor of an employee or annuitant to continue enrollment in a FEHBP plan in the event that the deceased had completed less than five years of creditable service.[44] FEHBP coverage was also extended to noncitizen employees whose permanent duty station was in the Panama Canal Zone.[45]

The Intergovernmental Personnel Act of 1970 (P.L. 91-648), January 5, 1971

The Act provided for the maintenance of FEHBP eligibility and coverage for federal employees who were assigned to state or local governments, and extended FEHBP coverage to state or local government employees who were assigned to an executive agency (where there would otherwise have been a loss of coverage in a group health benefits plan, the premium of which was paid in whole or in part by the state or local government).[46]

To Extend Civil Service Federal Employees Group Life Insurance and Federal Employees Health Benefits Coverage to United States Nationals Employed by the Federal Government (P.L. 93-160), November 27, 1973

The Act extended FEHBP coverage to otherwise eligible United States nationals employed by the federal government at permanent duty stations outside the United States and the Panama Canal Zone.

---

[42] Towers, Perrin, Forster, and Crosby, Inc. *Study of the Federal Employees Health Benefits Program*. Washington, 1988. p. 29.
[43] §1 of P.L. 91-418.
[44] §2 of P.L. 91-418.
[45] §3 of P.L. 91-418.
[46] §3373 of P.L. 91-648.

An Act to Increase the Contribution of the Government to the Costs of Health Benefits for Federal Employees, and for Other Purposes (P.L. 93-246), January 31, 1974

The Act increased the government's share of the FEHBP plan premium from 40% to 50% of the simple average of the big six premiums, for pay periods commencing in 1974.[47] A provision to increase the government's share to 60% of the big six average premiums for pay periods commencing in 1975 was also included in the Act. A maximum was set on the government's share so that it does not exceed 75% of the total premium amount for any one health plan.[48]

Additionally, health insurance plans participating in FEHBP were required to comply with OPM's decision in disputes regarding whether or not an individual was entitled to a health benefit.[49]

To Provide Access for all Duly Licensed Clinical Psychologists and Optometrists Without Prior Referral in the Federal Employee Health Benefits Program (P.L. 93-363), July 30, 1974

The Act provided that if a plan covers the services of licensed or certified optometrists or clinical psychologists, it cannot require referral or supervision by another practitioner as a condition for payment or reimbursement.[50]

To Amend Title 5, United States Code, to Grant Court Leave to Federal Employees When Called as Witnesses in Certain Judicial Proceedings, and for Other Purposes (P.L. 94-310), June 15, 1976

The amendments provided that government's share of health plan premiums for annuitants are to be paid from annual appropriations authorized for that purpose and made available until expended.[51]

To Amend Title 5, United States Code, to Restore Eligibility for Health Benefits Coverage to Certain Individuals Whose Survivor Annuities are Restored (P.L. 94-342), July 6, 1976

The Act provided that a surviving spouse covered by FEHBP who had his/her survivor annuity terminated due to remarriage is eligible to re-enroll in FEHBP if the survivor annuity is restored.

---

[47] The 40% government contribution rate was established by P.L. 91-418.

[48] §1 of P.L. 93-246. Previously, the government contribution was not to exceed 50% of the total premium amount for any one plan. See P.L. 89-504.

[49] §2 of P.L. 93-246.

[50] §1 of P.L. 93-363. The provision does not apply to group-practice prepayment plans, which are a type of comprehensive medical plan, as defined in the enacting FEHBP legislation (P.L. 86-382).

[51] §3 of P.L. 94-310.

To Amend Chapter 89 of Title 5, United States Code, to Establish Uniformity in Federal Employee Health Benefits and Coverage by Preempting Certain State or Local Laws Which are Inconsistent with such Contracts, and for Other Purposes (P.L. 95-368), September 17, 1978

The Act established uniformity in benefits and coverage under FEHBP by preempting certain state and local laws that were inconsistent with FEHBP contracts.

The Act provided certain protections to members of medically underserved populations.[52] Beginning January 1, 1980 and ending December 31, 1984, if a FEHBP contract provided or paid for the cost of a certain health service, the insurance carrier would be required to pay, up to the limits of its contract, for any health practitioner who is licensed by a state to provide that service if the recipient is a member of a medically underserved population.[53]

The Act also changed the requirement that barred employee organizations from appealing to sponsor a health benefit plan after January 1, 1964, permitting such organizations to apply between December 31, 1978 and January 1, 1980.

The Federal Employees Part Time Career Employment Act of 1978 (P.L. 95-437), October 10, 1978

The Act allowed part-time career employees and their dependents to access FEHBP coverage.[54] According to §3401(2) of U.S.C. Title 5, part-time career employment is employment consisting of a 16-32 hour work week, but does not include employment on a temporary or intermittent basis.

To Amend Subchapter m of Chapter 83 of Title 5, United States Code, to Provide that Employees who Retire After 5 Years of Service, in Certain Instances, May be Eligible to Retain their Life and Health Insurance Benefits, and for Other Purposes (P.L. 95-583), November 2, 1978

The Act reduced the length of *creditable service* required for an employee to continue FEHBP coverage in retirement from 12 years to five years (the 12-year requirement was established by P.L. 86-382). The Act *did not* change the requirement that in order for employees to continue FEHBP into retirement, they must be enrolled in a FEHBP plan for at least five years immediately prior to retirement, or enrolled from the earliest opportunity to do so (this requirement was established by P.L. 86-382).

---

[52] "Medically underserved population" as defined in §1302(7) of the Public Health Service Act (42 U.S.C. 300e-17).

[53] This provision does not apply to comprehensive medical plans.

[54] §4(c) of P.L. 95-437.

To Make Certain Technical and Clerical Amendments to Title 5, United States Code (P.L. 96-54), August 14, 1979

These amendments redefined "employee" for the purpose of FEHBP coverage to exclude the previous reference to the United States Commissioners (see P.L. 88-531).[55]

The Panama Canal Act of 1979 (P.L. 96-70), September 27, 1979

The Act redefined the term "employee" for the purposes of FEHBP eligibility to exclude individuals who were not citizens or nationals of the United States, and whose permanent duty station was outside the United States, *unless* the individual was an employee on September 30, 1979 at an executive branch agency, the United States Postal Service (USPS), or the Smithsonian Institution in the area which was then known as the Panama Canal Zone.[56]

To Amend Provisions of Chapters 83 and 89 of Title 5, United States Code, Which Relate to Survivor Benefits for Certain Dependent Children, and for Other Purposes (P.L. 96-179), January 2, 1980

The amendments eliminated the "lives with" requirement for a natural child to be covered by FEHBP and added a dependency requirement for all children to be covered under FEHBP.[57] It also redefined the term "medically underserved population" for the purpose of making benefit payments under FEHBP.[58]

The Tax Equity and Fiscal Responsibility Act of 1982 (P.L. 97-248), September 3, 1982

Effective January 1, 1983, the Act required federal employees to pay the Medicare hospital insurance tax. Requiring federal employees to pay the tax enabled federal employees to count their federal employment toward entitlement for premium-free benefits under Medicare Part A.[59] Prior to passing this Act, federal employment did not count toward eligibility for premium-free Part A, but federal employees could qualify for premium-free Part A based on private sector employment, if they were subject to the Medicare hospital insurance tax.

---

[55] §2(a)(52) of P.L. 96-54.

[56] §1209 of P.L. 96-70.

[57] §§1 and 2 of P.L. 96-179.

[58] §3 of P.L. 96-179.

[59] §§121 and 278 of P.L. 97-248. The hospital insurance tax is a payroll tax paid by most employees and employers, and it is used to help fund Medicare's Hospital Insurance Trust Fund, which pays for beneficiaries' Medicare Part A benefits. Individuals must pay into the system (i.e., incur the payroll tax) for 40 calendar quarters to become entitled to premium-free Part A benefits. Prior to enactment of P.L. 97-248, federal employees did not pay the Medicare hospital insurance tax and therefore their federal employment did not count toward the 40 calendar quarters required to obtain premium-free Part A benefits.

The Act also provided that Medicare payments are secondary for services provided to employees aged 65 to 69 (and their spouses aged 65 to 69) if covered under certain employer group health plans, including FEHBP.[60]

To Amend Title 5, United States Code, to Provide Training Opportunities for Employees Under the Office of the Architect of the Capitol and the Botanic Garden, and for Other Purposes (P.L. 97-346), October 15, 1982

The amendments required OPM to determine the difference between the amount of the government's share of health plan premiums for 1983 and the amount such contributions *would have been* if the two employee organizations included in the 1981 big six formula were included in the 1983 big six formula. The government was required to pay the difference into the contingency reserves of all FEHBP plans for 1983 in proportion to the number of enrollees in each plan.[61]

A Joint Resolution Making Further Continuing Appropriations for the Fiscal Year 1984 (P.L. 98-151), November 14, 1983

Funds appropriated by the continuing resolution were prohibited from being used to pay for abortions or administrative expenses for any FEHBP plan that provides benefits or coverage for abortions, except where the life of the woman would be endangered if the fetus were carried to term.[62] This was the first time an abortion-related provision was applied to FEHBP in an appropriations bill, and a similar provision has since been included in appropriations bills each year, with the exception of bills passed in the 103rd Congress.[63]

The Civil Service Retirement Spouse Equity Act of 1984 (P.L. 98-615), November 8, 1984

The Act extended eligibility for FEHBP coverage to former spouses of employed, retired, or separated federal employees. The former spouse must pay both the employee's and the government's share of the premium.[64]

---

[60] §116 of P.L. 97-248.

[61] §4 of P.L. 97-346. The enacting legislation (P.L. 86-382) requires that a certain percentage of the premiums paid to each plan by employees, annuitants, and the federal government is set aside to provide plans with contingency reserve funds. Funds from each plan's contingency reserves can be used to defray future premium increases, may be applied to reduce premium contributions of employees, annuitants, and the federal government, or may be used to increase the plan's benefits.

[62] §140 of P.L. 98-151.

[63] P.L. 103-123 and P.L. 103-329.

[64] §3 of P.L. 98-615.

An Act to Provide that Employee Organizations Ineligible to Participate in the FEHBP Solely Because Applications for Approval Must be Filed Before January 1, 1980, May Apply to Become so Eligible, and For Other Purposes (P.L. 99-53), June 17, 1985

The Act authorized the establishment of additional employee organization plans in FEHBP if the employee organization applied to OPM for plan approval within 90 days of enactment. It also specified the conditions required for plan approval.[65]

The Act also permitted certain disability annuitants who were later reemployed to enroll in a FEHBP plan if the annuitant had been enrolled in any such plan immediately prior to termination of employment.[66]

The Federal Employees Benefits Improvement Act of 1986 (P.L. 99-251), February 27, 1986

The Act allowed a new type of comprehensive medical plan, called a mixed model prepayment plan, to participate in FEHBP.[67] The plans are a combination of group practice prepayment plans and individual practice prepayment plans, which are two types of comprehensive medical plans recognized under FEHBP. Additionally, the requirement in the enacting legislation (P.L. 86-382) that group-practice prepayment plans must include physicians representing at least three major medical specialties was eliminated.[68]

The Act mandated studies to be undertaken by OPM regarding extending FEHBP contracting authority to health practitioners who were not currently covered, such as nurse midwives and chiropractors.[69] Contracting authority was also extended to clinical social workers, although health plans were permitted to require referral by a psychiatrist as a condition for reimbursement.[70]

The Act also expressed the sense of Congress that enrollees in FEHBP should receive adequate treatment for mental illness, alcoholism, and drug addiction.[71] In addition, OPM was directed to study the adequacy of the FEHBP information materials disseminated to employees during the open enrollment season.[72]

---

[65] §1 of P.L. 99-53.

[66] §3 of P.L. 99-53.

[67] §111 of P.L. 99-251.

[68] §102 of P.L. 99-251. Group-practice prepayment plans are a type of comprehensive medical plans under FEHBP.

[69] Sec. 108 of P.L. 99-251. OPM released this study, entitled, *A Study Relating to Expanding the Class of Health Practitioners Authorized to Receive Direct Payment or Reimbursement in Accordance with 5 U.S.C.*, 8902(k)(1) in March 1986.

[70] §105 of P.L. 99-251.

[71] §107 of P.L. 99-251.

[72] §109 of P.L. 99-251. OPM released this study, entitled *A Study of the Adequacy of Information Materials under the Federal Employees Health Benefits Program* in May 1986.

This Act gave OPM the authority to waive the five years of service requirement for individuals to have FEHBP coverage in retirement in cases of exceptional circumstances.[73] The Act provides for a three-week period during which enrollees may change or cancel their enrollment in the event that rates or benefits changed, a new plan is offered, or an existing plan is terminated. Enrollees were authorized to transfer enrollment at other times and under such circumstances as prescribed by OPM.[74]

The Consolidated Omnibus Budget Reconciliation Act of 1985 (P.L. 99-272), April 7, 1986

The Act required OPM to determine the minimum level of financial reserves which must be held by each carrier in order to ensure stable and efficient operation of the health plan. The Act set forth provisions regarding minimum amounts to be refunded, and the use of such amounts. Reserves held in excess of such minimum levels were to be returned to the Employees Health Benefits Fund. Beginning October 1, 1986, the United States Postal Service (USPS) was required to pay the government's share of the health plan premium for postal employees who first became annuitants because of retirement.[75] In addition, the Act provided that Medicare payments are secondary for services provided to employees aged 65 and older (which includes FEHBP or other certain employer group health plans).[76]

The Federal Employees' Retirement System Act of 1986 (P.L. 99-335), June 6, 1986

The Act provided FEHBP eligibility to individuals first employed by the District of Columbia government before October 1, 1987.[77]

The Intelligence Authorization Act for Fiscal Year 1987 (P.L. 99-569), October 27, 1986

The Act provided health benefits for certain former spouses of Central Intelligence Agency (CIA) employees.[78]

Treasury, Postal Services and General Government Appropriations Act, 1988 (P.L. 100-202), December 22, 1987

This Act added qualified clinical social workers to the group of non-physician providers to whom FEHBP enrollees must have direct access and who are entitled to receive payment by a FEHBP plan.[79]

---

[73] The five-year requirement was established in P.L. 95-583.
[74] §104 of P.L. 99-251.
[75] §15202 of P.L. 99-272.
[76] §9201 of P.L. 99-272.
[77] §207(c) of P.L. 99-353.
[78] §303 of P.L. 99-569.

The Omnibus Budget Reconciliation Act of 1987 (P.L. 100-203), December 22, 1987

The Act specified the amount ($160 million in FY1988 and $270 million in FY1989) of the contributions to be made by USPS to the Employees Health Benefits Fund to pay the government's share of the health plan premiums for certain USPS annuitants and survivor annuitants.[80]

The Foreign Relations Authorization Act, Fiscal Years 1988 and 1989 (P.L. 100-204), December 22, 1987

The Act provided FEHBP coverage for certain former spouses of employees or former employees of the Foreign Service.[81]

The Federal Employees' Retirement System Technical Corrections Act (P.L. 100-238), January 8, 1988

The Act declared that certain nonfederal employees who were eligible for FEHBP benefits were no longer entitled to such benefits after October 1, 1988.[82] However, the Act continued FEHBP coverage for employees of St. Elizabeth's Hospital who became District of Columbia employees due to the federal government's transfer of the hospital to the District of Columbia.[83]

Medicare Catastrophic Coverage Act of 1988 (P.L. 100-360), July 1, 1988

The Act included some provisions that affected FEHBP that were later repealed by the Medicare Catastrophic Coverage Repeal Act of 1989 (P.L. 101-234). They are described here for the purpose of providing a detailed account of Congress's interactions with FEHBP. Had it not been repealed, the Act would have (1) required OPM to reduce the rates charged to retirees participating in FEHBP who were also Medicare-eligible; (2) specified that the rates were to be reduced by the amount (prorated for each covered Medicare-eligible retiree) of the estimated cost of medical services and supplies which would have been incurred by FEHBP had certain provisions of the Act not been enacted;[84] (3) required OPM to submit a report to Congress by April 1, 1989 regarding changes to FEHBP that may be required in order to incorporate health benefit plans designed specifically for Medicare-eligible individuals and to improve the efficiency and effectiveness of the program; and (4) required OPM to submit a separate report to Congress by April 1, 1989 on the feasibility of adopting the National Association of Insurance

---

(...continued)

[79] §626, Title VI of P.L. 100-202.

[80] §6003 of P.L. 100-203.

[81] §832 of P.L. 100-204.

[82] §108 of P.L. 100-238.

[83] §109 of P.L. 100-238.

[84] §422 of P.L. 100-360. According to OPM, the premium reduction for 1989 would have been $3.10 per month for each Medicare eligible individual also participating in FEHBP had the provision related to reduced cost-sharing not been repealed.

Commissioners (NAIC) standards when providing Medicare supplemental health benefit plans under FEHBP.[85]

Federal Employees Health Benefits Amendments Act of 1988 (P.L. 100-654), November 14, 1988

The Act set forth provisions regarding the authority of OPM to impose debarment and other sanctions on health care providers convicted of illegal activities, including financial misconduct; neglect or abuse of patients; the unlawful manufacture, distribution, or dispensing of a controlled substance; and interference with an investigation or prosecution of any criminal offenses.

The Act also set time limits for OPM to initiate a debarment proceeding and prohibited providers without a valid license from participating in FEHBP. The Act authorized OPM to impose fines on providers who made false charges or claims in connection with providing health services or supplies.[86]

The Act created temporary continuation of FEHBP coverage (TCC) for federal employees. Effective in the 1990 contract year, TCC allows most separating employees and their families to maintain FEHBP coverage for up to 18 months after the date of separation.[87] TCC enrollees must pay the full premium, both the employee's and the government's share, for the plan they select, plus a 2% administrative charge. TCC is only available to employees separated from service for reasons other than gross misconduct, or for individuals no longer meeting unmarried dependent child requirements.[88]

The Act directed OPM to prescribe regulations to offer health benefits coverage to temporary federal employees who have completed one year of continuous service, with such employees paying the total premium amount.[89]

Office of Federal Procurement Policy Act Amendments of 1988 (P.L. 100-679), November 17, 1988

The Act provided that certain employees on the office staff of former Presidents or Vice Presidents are considered federal employees and are therefore eligible for FEHBP.[90]

---

[85] §424 of P.L. 100-360.

[86] §101 of P.L. 100-654.

[87] The Act allows some separating employees to maintain their temporary coverage for longer periods. Individuals who cease to meet the requirements for being considered a dependent child and certain former spouses may maintain TCC for 36 months.

[88] §201 of P.L. 100-654.

[89] §301 of P.L. 100-654.

[90] §13 of P.L. 100-679.

Relating to the Method by Which Government Contributions to the Federal Employees Health Benefits Program Shall be Computed for 1990 or 1991 if no Government-Wide Indemnity Benefit Plan Participates in that Year (P.L. 101-76), August 11, 1989

The Act adjusted the big six formula in response to Aetna's withdrawal from FEHBP.[91] The Act provided that for plan years 1990 and 1991, the government's share of FEHBP plans would be calculated by adjusting the Aetna high option premium for the previous year by the average percentage change in the remaining five plans included in the big six formula. The provisions of this Act would not apply if comprehensive reform legislation is enacted that amends FEHBP financing provisions. OPM must transmit recommendations to Congress for comprehensive FEHBP reform no later than 180 days after enactment.

Omnibus Budget Reconciliation Act of 1989 (P.L. 101-239), December 19, 1989

The Act required the USPS to pay the employer's (government's) share of FEHBP premiums for survivors of postal employees who retired on or after October 1, 1986, and survivors of postal employees who died on or after that date.[92]

Foreign Relations Authorization Act, Fiscal Years 1990 and 1991 (P.L. 101-246), February 16, 1990

The Act authorized FEHBP coverage for any former spouse who on February 14, 1981 was married to a former Foreign Service employee of the United States Information Agency or of the Agency for International Development if (1) the former employee retired from the Civil Service Retirement System on a date before his employing agency could legally participate in the Foreign Service Retirement System; (2) the marriage included at least five years during which the employee was assigned overseas; and (3) the former spouse is otherwise qualified for FEHBP.[93]

---

[91] The enacting FEHBP legislation (P.L. 86-382) provided that one of the plan types FEHBP could offer is one government-wide indemnity plan (with two levels). The Aetna Life Insurance Company offered the indemnity plan from the beginning of FEHBP through 1989, when Aetna decided it would no longer serve as the administrator of the plan. At the time, the government share of each plan's premium was the dollar amount equal to a percentage of the average cost of six plans (the big six), which included the indemnity plan. With Aetna's withdrawal from FEHBP and no insurance company filling Aetna's role as the administrator of the indemnity plan, the big six formula needed to be restructured.

[92] §4003 of P.L. 101-239.

[93] §146 of P.L. 101-246.

To Amend Title 5, United States Code, to Allow Federal Annuitants to Make Contributions for Health Benefits Through Direct Payments Rather than Through Annuity Withholdings if the Annuity is Insufficient to Cover the Required Withholdings, and for Other Purposes (P.L. 101-303), May 29, 1990

The Act allowed federal annuitants to pay health benefits premiums through direct payments rather than through annuity withholdings if the annuity is insufficient to cover the required withholdings.[94]

Omnibus Budget Reconciliation Act of 1990 (P.L. 101-508), November 5, 1990

The Act included a number of FEHBP-related reforms.[95] FEHBP plans must implement hospitalization cost containment measures, and FEHBP must improve cash management related to payments from a plan's contingency reserves. The Act exempted FEHBP plans from state premium taxes, and it extended the restructured big six formula created in P.L. 101-76 through plan year 1993 (originally the formula was to be used in plan years 1990 and 1991).

OPM, in consultation with HHS, is required to improve coordination between FEHBP and Medicare by creating a system that allows FEHBP plans to identify individuals who are entitled to Medicare benefits. Additionally, the Act applied Medicare payment limits to services that would be covered under Part A for retired FEHBP enrollees aged 65 and over who are not covered by Part A. This provision limited the amount that FEHBP pays for certain services for these individuals to the amount that Medicare would pay for the services.[96]

The Act also required the USPS to pay the government's share of FEHBP premiums for individuals who become annuitants because of retirement from employment with the USPS on or after July 1, 1971.[97] The amount paid by the USPS is prorated to reflect the total portion of federal service performed as a postal employee after June 30, 1971.[98]

Foreign Operations, Export Financing, and Related Programs Appropriations Act, 1991 (P.L. 101-513), November 5, 1990

The Act entitled U.S. hostages in Iraq, Kuwait, and those captured in Lebanon, and their family members, to FEHBP benefits while in hostage status and for 12 months thereafter, if they did not have other health insurance. Entitlement for these and certain other benefits (e.g., federal life insurance and pay) was subject to the availability of funds; the Act appropriated up to $10 million

---

[94] §1 of P.L. 101-303.

[95] §7002 of P.L. 101-508.

[96] The Medicare payment limits are not applied to services provided under comprehensive medical plans. Medicare has specific rules for payment of covered benefits, and all Medicare beneficiaries, including those who are also covered under FEHBP, are subject to the rules. For more information about the rules, see CRS Report RL30526, *Medicare Payment Policies*, coordinated by Paulette C. Morgan.

[97] Prior to enactment of P.L. 101-508, the USPS was required to pay the government share of premiums for postal service annuitants who retired on or after October 1, 1986.

[98] §§7102 and 7103 of P.L. 101-508.

for these benefits. The authority to obligate funds for this purpose expired six months after the date of enactment.[99]

Elimination of Post-1968 Service Prerequisite for Retirement Credit and Other Benefits (P.L. 101-530), November 6, 1990

The Act provided that post-1968 service by National Guard technicians is not a requirement for their eligibility for FEHBP benefits.[100]

Intelligence Authorization Act, Fiscal Year 1991 (P.L. 102-88), August 14, 1991

The Act amended the Central Intelligence Agency (CIA) Act of 1949 (P.L. 81-110) to provide that former spouses of certain CIA employees who are not eligible to enroll or continue enrollment in a FEHBP plan solely because of remarriage before age 55, may have their eligibility restored on the date such remarriage is dissolved by death, annulment, or divorce and may enroll in a FEHBP plan under certain circumstances.[101]

Legislative Branch Appropriations Act, 1992 (P.L. 102-90), August 14, 1991

This Act provided that employees of the Senate Employee Child Care Center are eligible for FEHBP coverage and may elect such coverage during the 31-day period beginning on the date of enactment or during FEHBP open enrollment periods thereafter.[102]

Treasury, Postal Service, and General Government Appropriations Act, 1993 (P.L. 102-393), October 6, 1992

Funds appropriated by the Act were prohibited from being used to implement changes to FEHBP that would affect Medicare beneficiaries.[103] Specifically, the Act restricted the use of appropriated funds to make certain changes to FEHBP. One restriction was to prevent OPM from requiring retired FEHBP enrollees who are eligible for Medicare benefits to pay the difference in out-of-pocket costs when using a nonparticipating Medicare provider (as compared to a participating Medicare provider).[104] The other restriction prevented OPM from eliminating the waiver of FEHBP plan coinsurance for prescription drugs used by Medicare-covered FEHBP enrollees. OPM intended to make both of these changes administratively for plan year 1993;[105] neither change was implemented due to the Act.

---

[99] §599C of P.L. 101-513.

[100] §§2 and 3 of P.L. 101-530. Previously, as established in P.L. 90-486, post-1968 service was a FEHBP eligibility requirement for National Guard technicians.

[101] §307 of P.L. 102-88.

[102] §311 of P.L. 102-90.

[103] §530 of P.L. 102-393.

[104] Most providers and practitioners are subject to limits on the amounts that they can bill Medicare beneficiaries for Medicare-covered services, and these limits are different according to a provider's contractual agreement with Medicare. For more information about "participating" and nonparticipating" providers within Medicare, see CRS Report R40425, *Medicare Primer*, coordinated by Patricia A. Davis.

[105] OPM administers FEHBP in accordance with the statue and its implementing regulations (5 CFR Part 89, and 48 (continued...)

National Defense Authorization Act for Fiscal Year 1993 (P.L. 102-484), October 23, 1992

The Act provided for the continuation of FEHBP benefits if the basis for such continuation is involuntary separation from a position in or under the Department of Defense due to a reduction in force. This provision applies to any individual whose temporary continued coverage (TCC) is based on a separation occurring on or after the date of enactment and before October 1, 1997 or February 1, 1998 (if specific notice of such separation was given to such individuals before October 1, 1997).[106] The Act limits the individual's payments for this coverage to no more than the required employee's share of premiums for such coverage and requires the agency that last employed the individual to pay for the remaining portion of the coverage.[107]

The Act directed the Secretary of Defense to conduct a comprehensive review of FEHBP in order to determine whether furnishing health care under a program similar to FEHBP to individuals eligible for health care programs provided by the Department of Defense would be more efficient and cost-effective.[108]

Omnibus Budget Reconciliation Act of 1993 (P.L. 103-66), August 10, 1993

The Act required most FEHBP plans to apply the Medicare Part B limitations on payments for physician services to benefits provided to any retired FEHBP enrollees aged 65 or older who do not participate in Medicare Part B.[109] The Act also required physicians and suppliers who accept Medicare payments to accept equivalent payment and cost-sharing from FEHBP as full payment for the services to the enrollees as described above. Physicians and suppliers who are non-participating physicians and suppliers in Medicare cannot impose charges that exceed the limiting charge with respect to the enrollees described above.[110]

The Act also provided for a temporary extension and modification of the restructured big six formula in the continued absence of a government-wide indemnity benefit plan.[111] The Act

---

(...continued)
CFR Chapter 16). While the statute establishes basic rules for the program, OPM is given wide authority in implementing regulations, contracting with plans, establishing benefits, and administering FEHBP. OPM's authority to generally administer FEHBP allows OPM to make certain changes to the program outside the legislative process. OPM introduced these particular changes in Carrier Letter 92-04, February 20, 1992.

[106] §4306 of P.L. 102-484.

[107] Section 8905a of Title 5 U.S.C. generally provides for temporary continued coverage (TCC) under FEHBP for individuals who were covered under FEHBP but no longer qualify due to either a change in employment or because the individual ceases to be an unmarried dependent child. Typically, the cost to the individual for TCC under FEHBP is the cost of both the employee's and the employer's share of benefits, in addition to an additional amount prescribed by OPM for administrative expenses (which cannot exceed 2% of the combined total of the employee's and the employer's shares).

[108] §723 of P.L. 102-484. The Secretary of Defense was required to submit to the Congressional defense committees a final report on the study no later than December 15, 1993.

[109] This provision does not apply to comprehensive medical plans under FEHBP. Medicare has specific rules for payment of covered benefits, and all Medicare beneficiaries, including those who are also covered under FEHBP, are subject to the rules. For more information about the rules, see CRS Report RL30526, *Medicare Payment Policies*, coordinated by Paulette C. Morgan.

[110] §11003 of P.L. 103-66. The "limiting charge" is defined in §1848(g) of the Social Security Act (SSA).

[111] §11005 of P.L. 103-66.

extended the formula developed in P.L. 101-76 for plan years 1990 and 1991 through plan year 1998, and modified the formula for plan years 1997 and 1998.

Treasury, Postal Service, and General Government Appropriations Act, 1994 (P.L. 103-123), October 28, 1993

This was the first appropriations act since fiscal year 1984 (P.L. 98-151) not to include the provision that restricts funding for abortion coverage in FEHBP plans.[112] The restriction on funding for abortion coverage was reinserted in the Treasury, Postal Service, and General Government Appropriations Act, 1996 (P.L. 104-52).

FEGLI Living Benefits Act, 1994 (P.L. 103-409), October 25, 1994

The Act allowed individuals covered under health benefit plans administered by the Office of the Comptroller of the Currency or the Office of Thrift Supervision (the Offices) to enroll in a FEHBP plan upon termination of the Offices' plans.[113] The Act provides that any period of enrollment under a health benefit plan administered by the Offices shall be deemed to be a period of enrollment under FEHBP.

Agriculture, Rural Development, Food and Drug Administration, and Related Agencies Appropriations Act, 1996 (P.L. 104-37), October 21, 1995

The Act allowed individuals covered under health benefit plans administered by the Farm Credit Administration to enroll in a FEHBP plan for coverage effective on and after September 30, 1995.[114] The Act also provided that any period of enrollment under a health benefit plan administered by the Farm Credit Administration prior to the enactment of the Act shall be deemed to be a period of enrollment under FEHBP.

Treasury, Postal Service, and General Government Appropriations Act, 1996 (P.L. 104-52), November 19, 1995

The Act reinstated the provision that prohibits appropriated funds from being available to pay for an abortion or the administrative expenses in connection with any health plan under FEHBP that provides any benefits or coverage for abortions, except where the life of the woman would be endangered if the fetus were carried to term. The provision is modified from the previous versions

---

[112] Additionally, the Treasury, Postal Service and General Government Appropriations Act, 1995 (P.L. 103-329), passed September 30, 1994, did not include a provision that restricted funding for abortion coverage in FEHBP plans.

[113] §5 of P.L. 103-409. Government agencies that have the authority to fix compensation (i.e., independent establishments as defined in §104 title 5 U.S.C. and government corporations as defined in §103 title 5 U.S.C.) generally also have the authority to offer health plans to their employees either in place of FEHBP or as an alternative to FEHBP. Prior to the enactment of P.L. 103-509, the Office of the Comptroller of the Currency and the Office of Thrift Supervision offered health plans as alternatives to FEHBP. For more information see GAO Report, "Independent Agencies Offering Their Own Health Plans," March 1989, http://www.gao.gov/assets/220/211072.pdf.

[114] §601 of P.L. 104-37. See footnote 103. Prior to the enactment of P.L. 104-37, the Farm Credit Administration offered its employees as health plan as an alternative to FEHBP.

to make an exception for pregnancy resulting from rape or incest.[115] This provision has been added each year to subsequent appropriations bills through the date of this report.

National Defense Authorization Act for Fiscal Year 1996 (P.L. 104-106), February 10, 1996

The Act changed how temporary continuation of FEHBP coverage (TCC) works for certain individuals. The Act allowed individuals who voluntarily separate from a surplus position in or under the Department of Defense or the Department of Energy, to continue coverage under FEHBP and be liable for no more than the employee's share of premiums to FEHBP.[116]

Omnibus Consolidated Appropriations Act, 1997 (P.L. 104-208), September 30, 1996

The Act required OPM to prescribe regulations under which surviving children, whose survivor annuity was terminated because of marriage and is later restored (because the marriage ends), may enroll in a FEHBP plan if such surviving child was covered by a FEHBP plan immediately before such annuity was terminated.[117]

The Secretary of Defense, in consultation with the HHS Secretary and the Director of OPM, was required to write a report containing recommendations for the establishment of a demonstration program.[118] The demonstration program would allow certain beneficiaries of Department of Defense health programs who are also entitled to Medicare Part A to enroll in a health plan offered through FEHBP.

Assisted Suicide Funding Restriction Act of 1997 (P.L. 105-12), April 30, 1997

The Act generally prohibited the use of federal funds for benefits and services related to assisted suicide, and it prohibited OPM from contracting with plans that include coverage for any of these benefits and services.[119]

Balanced Budget Act of 1997 (P.L. 105-33), August 5, 1997

The Act modified the formula for determining the government's share of FEHBP premiums.[120] The Act required OPM to determine the weighted average premium of all plans in FEHBP every year by October 1st.[121] This percentage is calculated separately for individual coverage and family

---

[115] §§ 524 and 525 of P.L. 104-52.

[116] Generally under TCC, an employee is responsible for both the employee's and the employer's (government's) share of the FEHBP premium, as well as an additional amount prescribed by OPM for administrative expenses (which cannot exceed 2% of the combined total of the employee's and the employer's shares). See P.L. 100-654.

[117] § 633 of P.L. 104-208.

[118] § 8129 of P.L. 104-208.

[119] §3 of P.L. 105-12.

[120] §7002 of P.L. 105-33.

[121] The weight given to each plan is required to be commensurate with the number of enrollees in such plan as of March 31st of the year in which the determination is made.

coverage, but the same formula is used. Under the Act, the biweekly government share of a FEHBP plan for an employee or annuitant is equal to 72% of the weighted average premium of all plans. (The Act maintained the provision enacted by P.L. 93-246 which provided that the biweekly government share cannot exceed 75% of any given plan's premium). This section of the Act took affect the first day of the contract year that began in 1999.

The Act also mandated that individuals enrolled in FEHBP are not eligible to enroll in a Medicare Medical Savings Account (MSA) plan[122] until OPM certifies to HHS that OPM has adopted policies that ensure that enrollment into such plans will not result in increased expenditures for the federal government.[123]

Strom Thurmond National Defense Authorization Act for Fiscal Year 1999 (P.L. 105-261) October 17, 1998

The Act directed the Secretary of Defense to enter into an agreement with the Director of OPM to conduct a demonstration project under which certain individuals eligible for Department of Defense health benefits were able to voluntarily enroll in health plans offered through FEHBP.[124] According to the Act, the demonstration project had to be conducted during three contract years under FEHBP; eligible beneficiaries were permitted to enroll during an open enrollment period for the year 2000; the project terminated December 31, 2002.

The Secretary of Defense and the Director of OPM were required to submit interim and final reports to Congress on project costs, effectiveness, and the feasibility of making the program permanent. The Comptroller General was also required to submit a report to Congress addressing the same issues as well as any limitations with respect to the data contained in the report as a result of the size and design of the demonstration project.

Federal Employees Health Care Protection Act of 1998 (P.L. 105-266), October 19, 1998

The Act provided for a number of largely administrative changes to FEHBP. OPM is required (rather than permitted) to debar health care providers[125] from FEHBP for certain fraudulent practices.[126] The Act modified the definition of a carrier under FEHBP from an "organization" to an "organization and an association of organizations or other entities described in this paragraph sponsoring a health benefits plan." It specified that the government-wide plan offered in FEHBP may be underwritten by participating affiliates licensed in each state. The Act also revised preemption provisions so that the terms of contract relating to the nature, provision, or extent of

---

[122] The definition of an MSA plan in P.L. 105-33 is a type of Medicare+Choice (now called Medicare Advantage) plan that provides reimbursement for items and services only after the enrollee incurs expenses equal to the amount of the annual deductible.

[123] §1851 of P.L. 105-33.

[124] §721 of P.L. 105-261.

[125] A "health care provider" is defined in §8902a of title 5 U.S.C as a "physician, hospital, or other individual or entity which furnishes health care services or supplies."

[126] §2 of P.L. 105-266.

coverage or benefits under FEHBP shall supersede and preempt any state or local law, or any regulation issued by a state or local entity, which relates to health insurance or plans.[127]

OPM is required to encourage carriers that enter into contractual arrangements to obtain discounts from providers for health care services or supplies to seek assurance that the conditions for such discounts are fully disclosed to the providers who grant them.[128] The Act set forth provisions for the readmission of certain plans that have discontinued their participation in FEHBP, and the treatment of the contingency reserves of such discontinued plans.[129] Plans under FEHBP are allowed to provide direct access, direct payment, or reimbursement to specified licensed health care providers.[130]

The Act provided that individuals enrolled in Federal Deposit Insurance Corporation (FDIC) health plans or health plans available to the Board of Governors of the Federal Reserve System may enroll in FEHBP plans when the FDIC and Federal Reserve plans terminate.[131] The Act also provided that any period of enrollment in a health benefits plan administered by FDIC or the Federal Reserve before the termination of such plan (January 2, 1999) is deemed to be a period of enrollment in FEHBP.

District of Columbia Courts and Justice Technical Corrections Act of 1998 (P.L. 105-274), October 21, 1998

The Act provided that Public Defender Service employees should be treated as federal employees for eligibility for health insurance under FEHBP, compensation for work injuries, retirement, and life insurance.[132]

Omnibus Consolidated and Emergency Supplemental Appropriations Act, 1999 (P.L. 105-277), October 21, 1998

The Act required all FEHBP plans to cover contraceptives, with the exception of a few specified plans[133] and any other existing or future plan that objects to such coverage on the basis of

---

[127] This Act revises language relating to preemption of state laws that was originally crafted in P.L. 95-368.

[128] §5 of P.L. 105-266.

[129] §6 of P.L. 105-266.

[130] §8 of P.L. 105-266.

[131] §4 of P.L. 105-266. Government agencies that have the authority to fix compensation (i.e., independent establishments as defined in §104 title 5 U.S.C. and government corporations as defined in §103 title 5 U.S.C.) generally also have the authority to offer health plans to their employees either in place of FEHBP or as an alternative to FEHBP. Prior to the enactment of P.L. 105-266, the Federal Deposit Insurance Corporation and the Board of Governors of the Federal Reserve System offered its employees a health plan as an alternative to FEHBP. For more information see GAO Report, "Independent Agencies Offering Their Own Health Plans," March 1989, http://www.gao.gov/assets/220/211072.pdf.

[132] §7 of P.L. 105-274.

[133] The plans specifically excluded from the requirement for coverage of contraceptives in the appropriations bills are: Providence Health Plan; Personal Care's HMO; Care Choices; OSF Health Plans, Inc.; Yellowstone Community Health Plan. According to OPM, in contract year 2012, none of these excepted plans still participated in FEHBP, and no plan had a religious exception from providing contraceptive coverage.

religious beliefs.[134] As of the date of this report, this provision has been renewed each year in subsequent appropriations bills.

Veterans Millennium Health Care and Benefits Act (P.L. 106-117), November, 30, 1999

The Act changed how temporary continuation of FEHBP coverage (TCC) works for certain individuals. The Act allowed certain individuals to continue coverage under FEHBP and be liable for no more than the employee's share of premiums to FEHBP,[135] specifically those: (1) who are involuntarily separated from a position in or under the Department of Veteran Affairs due to a reduction in force or certain staffing readjustments; or (2) who are voluntarily or involuntarily separated from certain Department of Energy positions.

National Defense Authorization Act for Fiscal Year 2000 (P.L. 106-65), October 5, 1999

The Act required the Secretary of Defense to compare the case management program of the Department of Defense and the case management coverage offered by at least 10 of the most subscribed plans in FEHBP (five of which must be managed care organizations).[136] The Act also required the Secretary of Defense to submit a report that includes a comparison of health care coverage under TRICARE to coverage available under FEHBP.[137] The comparison must include, but not be limited to, a comparison of cost sharing requirements, overall costs to beneficiaries, covered benefits, and exclusions from coverage.

Federal Employees Health Benefits Children's Equity Act of 2000 (P.L. 106-394), October 30, 2000

The Act mandated that an employee who is required by court or administrative order to provide health insurance coverage for a dependent child must do so under FEHBP if the employee cannot provide documentation of other health insurance coverage for the child.[138] If the employee is no longer enrolled in FEHBP, the employing federal agency is directed to enroll the employee in a family plan that provides the lower level of coverage under the Service Benefit Plan (if the employee fails to enroll and cannot provide documentation of other coverage for the child.)[139] If the employee has individual coverage under FEHBP, the employee is authorized to change to family coverage. If the employee does not change his or her coverage, the employing federal agency is directed to change the enrollment of the employee to family coverage either in the plan

---

[134] §656 of P.L. 105-277.

[135] Generally under TCC, an employee is responsible for both the employee's and the employer's (government's) share of the FEHBP premium, as well as an additional amount prescribed by OPM for administrative expenses (which cannot exceed 2% of the combined total of the employee's and the employer's shares). See P.L. 100-654.

[136] §703 of P.L. 106-65.

[137] §717 of P.L. 106-65.

[138] §2 of P.L. 106-394.

[139] According to §8903 title 5 U.S.C., OPM may contract with one "Service Benefit Plan" under FEHBP, which is a government-wide fee-for-service plan offering two levels of benefits. Blue Cross Blue Shield has been the Service Benefit Plan offered in FEHBP since the program's inception.

in which the employee is currently enrolled, or the lower level of coverage under the nationally-available Service Benefit Plan.

Floyd D. Spence National Defense Authorization Act for Fiscal Year 2001 (P.L. 106-398), October 30, 2000

The Act directed the Secretary of Defense to conduct a study comparing Department of Defense health programs with plans under Medicare and FEHBP in the areas of coverage and reimbursement for physical, speech, and occupational therapies.[140]

District of Columbia Appropriations Act, 2001 (P.L. 106-522), November 22, 2000

The Act allowed certain employees of the District of Columbia to be treated as federal employees for purposes relating to certain federal programs, including FEHBP. These employees are eligible for benefits under FEHBP, and the District of Columbia is required to contribute to FEHBP premiums at the same rates as federal agencies.[141]

National Defense Authorization Act for Fiscal Year 2002 (P.L. 107-107), December 28, 2001

The Act authorized employing agencies to pay both the employee's and employer's (government's) share of premiums for health care coverage under FEHBP for certain reservists who are enrolled in a FEHBP plan and are called to active duty in support of a contingency operation.[142]

The Act also directed the Comptroller General to carry out a study of the health benefit needs of members of the reserve components of the Armed Forces and the National Guard and their families with an assessment of the cost and effectiveness of various options, including providing FEHBP coverage to all members of the reserve components of the Armed Forces and the National Guard and their families.[143]

To Amend Title 5, United States Code, to Allow Certain Catch-up Contributions to the Thrift Savings Plan to be Made by Participants Age 50 or Over (P.L. 107-304), November 27, 2002

The Act allowed beneficiaries of a health benefits plan administered by the Overseas Private Investment Corporation (OPIC) to obtain FEHBP coverage when OPIC-administered plans terminate.[144] Any period of enrollment under an OPIC-administered plan before the effective date

---

[140] §762 of P.L. 106-398.
[141] §145 of P.L. 105-522.
[142] §519 of P.L. 107-107.
[143] §721 of P.L. 107-107.
[144] §4 of P.L. 107-304.

of the Act is to be considered a period of enrollment in FEHBP for the purposes of administration of FEHBP coverage.[145]

Bob Stump National Defense Authorization Act for Fiscal Year 2003 (P.L. 107-314), December 2, 2002

The Act extended certain individuals' access to temporary continuation of FEHBP coverage (TCC). The Act extended a provision that allows individuals who are involuntarily separated from military service, or voluntarily separated from a surplus position in the Departments of Defense or Energy due to a reduction in force, to temporarily continue coverage under FEHBP and only pay the employee's share of premiums.[146] The extension applies to individuals separated through FY2005 (at the time the Act was passed, the provision applied to individuals separated through FY2002).

State Justice Institute Reauthorization Act of 2004 (P.L. 108-372), October 25, 2004

The Act extended FEHBP coverage to State Justice Institute employees who began employment on or after October 1, 1988.[147]

Ronald W. Reagan National Defense Authorization Act for Fiscal Year 2005 (P.L. 108-375), October 28, 2004

The Act provided for the temporary continuation of FEHBP coverage for up to 24 months for a federal employee who is (1) currently enrolled in the FEHBP; and (2) is a member of the reserve component of the Armed Forces and called or ordered to active duty in support of a contingency operation and serves on such duty for more than 30 consecutive days.[148] Prior to the Act, temporary continuation of coverage (TCC) was generally provided to employees and their family members who voluntarily and involuntarily lost FEHBP coverage, but TCC was not explicitly provided for federal employees who were called to active duty as members of the reserve component of the armed forces.

---

[145] Government agencies that have the authority to fix compensation (i.e., independent establishments as defined in §104 title 5 U.S.C. and government corporations as defined in §103 title 5 U.S.C.) generally also have the authority to offer health plans to their employees either in place of FEHBP or as an alternative to FEHBP. Prior to the enactment of P.L. 107-304, the Overseas Private Investment Corporation offered a health plan to its employees as an alternative to FEHBP. For more information see GAO Report, "Independent Agencies Offering Their Own Health Plans," March 1989, http://www.gao.gov/assets/220/211072.pdf.

[146] §1103 of P.L. 107-314. Generally under TCC, an employee is responsible for both the employee's and the employer's (government's) share of the FEHBP premium, as well as an additional amount prescribed by OPM for administrative expenses (which cannot exceed 2% of the combined total of the employee's and the employer's shares). See P.L. 100-654.

[147] §3 of P.L. 108-372.

[148] §1101 of P.L. 108-375.

Intelligence Authorization Act for Fiscal Year 2005 (P.L. 108-487), December 23, 2004

The Act authorized the Director of the Central Intelligence Agency (CIA) to take certain actions to protect the unauthorized disclosure of intelligence operations, the identities of undercover intelligence officers, and intelligence sources and methods. In doing this, the Director of the CIA, among other things, may establish and administer a nonofficial cover employee health insurance program for designated employees and their families.[149] A designated employee that participates in this program cannot simultaneously participate in FEHBP. However, a designated employee participating in the nonofficial program may convert to coverage under FEHBP at any time deemed appropriate by the Director of the CIA.

Federal Employee Dental and Vision Benefits Enhancement Act of 2004 (P.L. 108-496), December 23, 2004

The Act directed OPM to submit a report to Congress describing and evaluating options whereby health insurance coverage under FEHBP could be made available to unmarried dependent children under 25 years of age who are enrolled as full-time students at institutions of higher education.[150]

An Act to amend chapter 89 of title 5, United States Code, to make individuals employed by the Roosevelt Campobello International Park Commission eligible to obtain Federal health insurance (P.L. 110-74), August 9, 2007

The Act allowed U.S. citizens employed by the Roosevelt Campobello International Park Commission to be eligible to obtain health insurance under FEHBP.[151]

An Act to provide for certain Federal employee benefits to be continued for certain employees of the Senate Restaurants after operations of the Senate Restaurants are contracted to be performed by a private business concern, and for other purposes (P.L. 110-279), July 17, 2008

The Act authorized the continued coverage of federal benefits, including FEHBP, for certain employees of Senate restaurants who are employees of the Architect of the Capitol after operations of the Senate Restaurants are contracted to be performed by a private business concern.[152]

---

[149] §402(e) of P.L. 108-487.
[150] §6 of P.L. 108-496.
[151] §1 of P.L. 110-74.
[152] §1 of P.L. 110-279.

National Aeronautics and Space Administration Authorization Act of 2008 (P.L. 110-422), October, 15, 2008

The Act specified requirements related to temporary continuation of coverage (TCC) under FEHBP for NASA employees terminated from the Space Shuttle Program; involuntarily separated from a position due to a reduction-in-force, declination of a directed reassignment, or transfer of function; or a voluntary separation from a surplus position. The Act required that if such an employee is receiving TCC under FEHBP, then the employee is not liable for more than the employee's share of the premium for the same health benefits plan and level of benefits. The Act requires NASA to pay the remaining share of the premium required under FEHBP.[153]

The requirement for such TCC is applicable to individuals whose continued coverage is based on a separation occurring on or after enactment of this section and before December 31, 2010.

Patient Protection and Affordable Care Act (P.L. 111-148, as amended), March 23, 2010

Beginning in 2014, Members of Congress and congressional staff may only enroll in health plans created under ACA, or offered through an exchange. Congressional staff, for the purpose of this requirement, will be limited to those part-and full-time employees who are employed by the official office of a Member of Congress (i.e., in a "personal office").[154]

The Act allowed eligible Indian tribes, tribal organizations, and urban Indian organizations to purchase FEHBP for their tribal employees. The tribe or tribal organization is responsible for paying the government's share of the premium, at a minimum, with the enrollee paying the remaining share. The Act only allows tribes and tribal organizations to purchase this coverage for employees; coverage is not available to their annuitants.[155]

The Act required that adult children up to age 26 may remain/enroll on their parent's health insurance plan.[156] This provision generally applies to all types of health insurance coverage, not just coverage offered though FEHBP. As a result of extending dependent coverage to age 26, temporary continued coverage (TCC) is available for three years when the child ages out of FEHBP at age 26. Similarly, the opportunity for certain disabled children to remain on their parent's plan is tied to age 26. If a disability affected a child prior to age 26, the child may remain a dependent on his/her parent's plan indefinitely.

---

[153] §615 of P.L. 110-422. Generally, TCC enrollees pay the full premium, both the employee's and the employer's share, plus a 2% administrative charge. See P.L. 100-654.

[154] §1312 of P.L. 111-148.

[155] §157 of the Indian Health Care Improvement Reauthorization and Extension Act of 2009 (S. 1790) as enacted by §10221(a) of P.L. 111-148.

[156] §1001 of P.L. 111-148 adding §2714 to the Public Health Service Act, as amended by §2301 of P.L. 111-152.

Author Contact Information

Annie L. Mach
Analyst in Health Care Financing
amach@crs.loc.gov, 7-7825

Ada S. Cornell
Information Research Specialist
acornell@crs.loc.gov, 7-3742

www.ingramcontent.com/pod-product-compliance
Lightning Source LLC
Chambersburg PA
CBHW081244180526
45171CB00005B/533